Simple Fitness

For Your Body, Mind, and Spirit

Simple Fitness

For Your Body, Mind, and Spirit

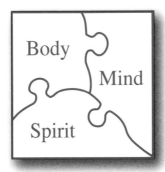

Body

Mind

Spirit

Joyce Meek Yates, Ed.D.

Amanda Gladney Conrad

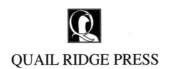

QUAIL RIDGE PRESS

Library of Congress Cataloging-in-Publication Data

Yates, Joyce Meek
    Simple fitness : for your body, mind, and spirit / Joyce Meek Yates
    & Amanda Gladney Conrad.
        p. cm.
    Includes bibliographical references.
    ISBN 1-893062-53-8
      1. Physical fitness. 2. Exercise. 3. Health. I. Conrad, Amanda Gladney.
    II. Title.

    RA781.C593 2003
    613.7—dc21   2003046729

9 8 7 6 5 4 3 2 1

ISBN 1-893062-53-8

Design by Cynthia Clark.
Printed in the United States of America.

QUAIL RIDGE PRESS
P. O. Box 123 • Brandon, MS 39043 • 1-800-343-1583
email: info@quailridge.com • www.quailridge.com

Dedication

This book is dedicated to
all who seek direction in taking
responsibility for their health and,
in effect, control of their lives;
and to those who live with disease
or infirmity that could be
avoided by taking charge of
controllable risk factors.

Table of Contents

Introduction

"Look to your health; and if you have it, praise God and value it next to conscience; for health is the second blessing that we mortals are capable of, a blessing money can't buy."

– Izaak Walton

At any given time, millions of Americans are striving to improve some aspect of their life. Sometimes this aspect is physical, sometimes it is emotional, and sometimes it is spiritual. Oftentimes it is some combination of the three. Setting goals for yourself, working on improvements, and feeling great about these accomplishments is essential to your well-being.

We have worked with various people in many different settings—from the perfectly healthy college student, to senior citizens, to cardiac rehabilitation patients, to the average public, and everything in between. A common goal among them all is to improve health and wellness. But, with so much conflicting infor-mation on the market, it is easy to get helpless-ly lost in any effort to pursue a healthy lifestyle. Our goal is to help you understand what you need to do by focusing on the simple. *Simple Fitness for Your Body, Mind, and Spirit* will not bog you down with intimidating information, and it will not make you feel defeated by tedious, rule-laden programs. In *Simple Fitness,* we have compiled well-established, research-proven, concise, common sense ideas into a format that is easy-to-read, easy-to-learn, and easy-to-follow. This book will help you understand the basic concepts of total body fitness and give you ideas on how to apply these concepts to your daily life.

Six areas of health are addressed in *Simple Fitness for Your Body, Mind, and Spirit:* physical health, nutritional health, social health, intellectual health, emotional health, and spiritual health. Development of all six of these key areas of fitness is necessary in achieving long-term success in healthy lifestyle management. Improvements in one of these areas will strengthen the health of the other components.

To get a visual grasp of how these various health components work together to influence your vitality, compare the health of your whole body to that of a three-piece puzzle. Each piece stands for a portion of health and wellness—mind, body, and spirit. Separately they have little or no function, but when fitted together, they become one. If the mind is calm, the spirit is peaceful, and the body is fit, then synergy occurs among the whole. If you really want to feel good, you cannot leave out any piece of the puzzle. You must develop all three aspects being sure not to ignore the spiritual aspect. Throughout the Bible the message is clear that for abundant life through Christ, you must embrace an existence of service, self-sacrifice, and love. With the strength of the Christian spirit and a heart for the Lord, changes are made within the human soul that allow perspectives and priorities to be humbled and changed. God invites us to live the abundant life.

We don't pretend to have the "magic wand" that controls your will to make the important decisions that guarantee successful living and wellness. We do, however, give you the formula that will help you attain a healthier degree of optimal living, if you simply follow the principles and practices suggested in *Simple Fitness for Your Body, Mind, and Spirit.*

Simple Fitness will help you understand the basic concepts of a healthy lifestyle by giving you ideas that you can use to apply these concepts to your daily life. We have seen it work numerous times. When you start focusing on the small, simple solutions that can be worked into your daily life, you will begin to understand that a healthy lifestyle is definitely in reach.

Just try it. Rather than a before and after picture of traditional fitness or weight loss programs, have a before and after "feeling." Right now, before you go any further into the book, write down how you feel. Include how you feel about your body, how you feel in your daily routine, how you feel spiritually. Include your feelings on all aspects of health and life in general. Put these thoughts and feelings aside. Now, continue with the book. Whether you read it front to back, a page a day, a section a week, or even if you are just picking it up and reading where the page opens, take what you read to heart and start applying it to your life. Let each reading guide you to improvements in each aspect of your health. Let these improvements build upon each other, leading you to a more fulfilled and healthy life. In a month, again write down how you feel. Compare it to the first time you recorded these feelings. You'll achieve greater confidence as the results become more noticeable.

We hope *Simple Fitness for Your Body, Mind, and Spirit,* with its researched, time-tested facts and easy suggestions of principles and practices, will intrigue and energize you to seek your optimal quality of life. After all, isn't that what we all want—to feel good and live each day simply but to its fullest?

J.M.Y./A.G.C.

Simple Fitness
For Your Body

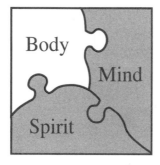

*B*efore you begin an exercise program, have a thorough medical examination. This is especially important for people who live with chronic disease or other risk factors and for males over 40 and females over 50.

Practice

Get medical clearance today. Make an appointment with your family physician. Have all necessary medical screenings performed. Have your cholesterol and blood pressure checked.

*I*n the 1996 report Physical Activity and Health, *the Surgeon General suggests individuals participate in a moderate amount of physical activity on most, if not all, days of the week to improve health benefits.*

Practice

Walking is an example of moderate exercise. Start slowly. Try to build pace and time by walking a 20- to 25-minute mile when you begin your walking exercise program. After two weeks at this pace, try to shorten your time by three to five minutes. Periodically decrease your time by increasing your walking pace. Make a 15-minute mile your goal.

*B*enefits of physical activity include:
- *Lower incidence of cardiovascular disease*
- *Lower incidence of diabetes*
- *Lower incidence of osteoporosis*
- *Lower risk for cancer (especially colon and breast)*
- *Lower risk for hypertension*
- *Reduced stress*
- *More energy*
- *Less body fat*
- *Enhanced immune system*
- *More efficient metabolism*
- *Stronger posture*
- *Improved sleep*
- *Regular digestion and excretion*

Practice

Pick at least five of the bulleted benefits above that you want to claim right now. Make these benefits your personal fitness goals. Remind yourself of these goals by posting them where you can easily see them—by your bed, on the refrigerator, or in your planner.

If you have trouble remembering just how much exercise you need, think of the acronym F.I.T.—Frequency, Intensity, and Time.

Practice

Let F.I.T. be your guide to ensure an improvement in cardiovascular health and other disease risk factors.

F = Frequency
How often? Exercise three to five days a week.

I = Intensity
How hard? Work out hard enough to get your heart rate in your target heart rate range (see page 22).

T = Time
How long? Work out for a minimum of 20 minutes. As your fitness improves, increase your workout time up to an hour.

*T*he duration of the activity you perform is more important than the activity you choose.

Practice

Begin with low intensity activity and build week by week until you progress to moderate activity. Then, choose high intensity workouts, if you prefer.

If you are satisfied with **low intensity exercise,** perform them at least five to seven times weekly for 30 minutes or more. Low intensity activity includes walking, stretching, easy housework or light yard work and any activity that does not tax the cardiorespiratory system.

Moderate activity promotes high levels of health benefits. As reported by the Surgeon General's report, for maximum health benefits, regular moderate activity requires a total of 30 minutes or more

(continued on next page)

(continued from previous page)
per day for a frequency of at least five days a week. Moderately intense activity includes stair climbing, moderate yard work, brisk walking, moderate house cleaning, team games, and other similar activities. You must perform at least 20 minutes of vigorous activity each session three days a week or more to achieve a maximum health benefit.

Vigorous or high intensity activity includes running, jogging, aerobics, swimming, individual sports and biking. Circuit training on exercise equipment and strength training may be termed vigorous depending on the amount of repetitions and weight being used.

*F*lexibility is an important aspect of fitness.

Practice

Suggested stretches: 1) Sit on the floor, straighten your back with your legs extended in front of you. Reach for your toes without bending your knees. Count to five, release, then repeat. 2) In a standing position, place your feet shoulder-width apart, extend your right arm up and lean to the left side as far as you can go and count to five. Release and repeat. Continue with opposite arm and lean to your right side. It is easier to stretch after or during a warm bath or shower. Make bath time a routine stretching time since the muscle groups are warmed by the temperature of the water.

*E*xercise *helps the heart and respiratory system to work more efficiently.*

Practice

Don't get caught in one position for long periods of time. Do squats while talking on the phone. Take the stairs instead of the elevator. Park at the back of the parking lot. Stretch every hour. Contract abdominal muscles for five seconds and release at each traffic light; repeat. Ride your bicycle to destinations instead of driving your car. (Be sure to wear your bicycle helmet.) Get moving!

Your target heart rate zone is the range between 60% and 80% of your maximum heart rate. Working within this zone gives you the maximum health and fat-burning benefits from your cardiovascular activity.

Practice

Exercise three to five times a week for at least 20 to 30 minutes at your target heart rate in order to have a cardio-respiratory effect.

To determine if you are working within your zone, locate your radial artery at the side of your wrist with your index finger and count the beats for 15 seconds. This result should be within the minimum and maximum training heart rate values listed on the next page:

(continued from previous page)

AGE	TARGET HEART RATE	15-SECOND COUNT
20-24	120-160	30-40
25-29	117-156	29-39
30-34	114-152	29-38
35-39	111-148	28-37
40-44	108-144	27-36
45-49	105-140	26-35
50-54	102-136	26-34
55-59	99-132	25-33
60-64	96-128	24-32
65+	90-124	23-31

Physical Health

he leading causes of death in the United States are: first, heart disease; second, cancer; third, strokes. All three are greatly affected by lifestyle choices.

Practice

Adopt a healthy lifestyle and refuse to become a part of this statistic. For a healthy heart, exercise at least 30 minutes most days and strength train at least two days a week. Routine exercise is also related to lower incidence of colon and other cancers.

For example, perform any of the following activities for 30 minutes:
- Walk two miles
- Cycle
- Work out to an exercise tape
- Play singles tennis
- Swim
- Dance

Physical Health

*P*hysical Activity Steps

Moderate Intensity Activites

30 minutes daily (combined)

Walking, Housework, Yard work, Parking the car and walking instead, Taking the stairs instead of the elevator, Moderate intensity swimming

Aerobic Activites

3-5 days a week for 20-30 minutes at target heart rate*

Jogging, Running, High intensity walking, Aerobic and work-out videos, Basketball, Soccer

*See page 22

Strength Training Activites

2-3 days a week (alternate major muscle groups)

Any weight-bearing activity, Push-ups, Sit-ups, Curls, Exercise machines

Sedentary Activites

Sparingly

Watching TV, Surfing internet, Riding in car or sitting for long periods of time

Practice

If you are currently sedentary, gradually increase the amount of moderate-intensity activities. If you are moderately active, begin a formal exercise program that includes each component of fitness.

*T*hirty to seventy percent of people who start exercise programs drop out within six months. Don't become part of the statistic.

Practice

Adopt exercise that can be a part of your daily routine and can be performed conveniently near home or work. Be careful not to set your fitness goal too high from the beginning. Review your guidelines and be realistic. Seek the support of family and friends. Participate in an activity you enjoy and you will have greater success.

Research has revealed that people who exercise first thing in the morning tend to stay with their exercise routines more readily.

Practice

Wake up and get moving. Make exercise a morning routine just like brushing your teeth. You will feel better the rest of the day, and you will give your metabolism a jump start!

*R*ocking chairs are good for the back. The gentle, alternating actions of the abdominal and back muscles prevent the inactive postures that often lead to back pain.

Practice

Place a rocking chair in the perfect, serene spot for your relaxation. Work those back muscles and meditate on pleasant thoughts. Everyone needs a break. Take time out to relax and rock.

If you occasionally feel faint when suddenly rising from a lying or seated position, it could be caused by a temporary drop of blood pressure.

Practice

Be careful. Before standing, stretch your legs and flex your feet while tightening your stomach muscles. This circulates the blood that has collected in your legs. Consult your doctor if faintness persists.

*P*eople who exercise regularly benefit emotionally, socially, and psychologically.

Practice

Exercise for the release of stress. You will reap the benefits immediately by experiencing less anxiety and becoming somewhat protected from the dangerous physical effects of stress. You will also experience less anxiety. Exercise helps or lessens the effects of depression and is beneficial for good mental health.

$\mathcal{B}$ody Mass Index (BMI) is an index of a person's weight in relation to height that closely correlates with the proportion of your body that consists of fat.

BMI = Weight (pounds) ÷ Height (inches)^2 X 705

Note: To obtain height squared, multiply the number (in inches) to itself. For example 5 feet = 60 inches X 60 = 3,600.

Practice

In order to decrease your risk of certain health problems and improve your overall well-being, aim for a BMI of 19-24.9. A balanced diet and exercise program will help you achieve this range.

*G*eneral *Activity Guide for Calorie Burning*

ACTIVITY	CALORIES BURNED PER HOUR
Sleeping	65
Watching TV	80
Driving Car	100
Dishwashing	135
Bowling	190
Walking (25 min/mile)	225
Dancing	250
Strength Training	300
Swimming	300
Gardening	390
Tennis	425
Soccer	600
Jogging	655
Running	800

Practice

Use this as a guide for burning more calories than you consume if weight-loss is your goal.

Weight training helps keep the skeleton in proper alignment, provides strength in sports and activities, helps prevent osteoporosis, lessens injury to your back and legs, and provides toning for large muscle groups.

Practice

If you use light weights, do 8 to 12 repetitions of each exercise. If you use heavier weights, use a lower sequence of repetitions. Your own muscle groups can act as weights in such exercises as crunches or push-ups. Incorporate weight training into your weekly fitness routine.

Energy Balance Equation

The central concept related to weight control is found in the energy balance equation:

- *If caloric intake is **equal to** expenditure, then energy balance exists—no change in weight occurs.*

- *If caloric intake is **greater than** caloric expenditure, then positive energy balance exists—weight gain occurs.*

- *If caloric intake is **less than** caloric expenditure, then negative energy balance exists—weight loss occurs.*

Practice

Decide which energy balance equation is right for you. (See page 32 for calorie burning suggestions.)

One pound of fat is equal to 3,500 calories. If you consume 3,500 more calories than you expend, you will gain one pound of fat. If you expend 3,500 more calories than you consume, you will lose a pound.

Practice

If weight loss is your goal, you can safely lose weight by having a 500-calorie deficit per day. Decrease your caloric intake by 250 calories and increase your activity level by at least 250 calories each day (see page 32). (500 calories/day x 7 day/week = 3,500 calories)

*D*etermine how many calories your body needs each day. When you have reached your limit, stop.

Practice

Determine your **Resting Metabolic Rate** (RMR) to learn how many calories you need in a day.

Step 1: Change your weight in pounds to kilograms: Your weight in pounds ÷ 2.2 = Your weight in kilograms

Step 2: Change your height in inches to centimeters: Your height in inches X 2.54 = Your height in centimeters

Step 3: Determine how much energy you expend at rest by inserting your answers to Steps 1 and 2 into the appropriate formula (based on gender). The answer you get is the number of calories your body needs at rest.

(continued on next page)

(continued from previous page)

Women's Resting Energy Expenditure
= 655 + 9.56 X weight in kilograms +
1.85 X height in centimeters – 4.68
X age in years

Men's Resting Energy Expenditure
= 6.5 + 13.75 X weight in kilograms
+ 5.0 X height in centimeters – 6.78
X age in years

Step 4: To figure out how many calories you need a day based on your activity level, multiply the answer from Step 3 with the appropriate number that correlates with your activity level.

Very inactive: 1.3
Most normally active persons:
    1.5-1.75
Extremely active persons: 2.0-2.4

This answer is an estimation of how many calories are needed for you to maintain your current weight.

Nutritional Health

*F*ive Basic Diet Planning Principles

1. **Adequacy**—*Make sure your diet keeps you energized and supplied with nutrients.*

2. **Calorie Control**—*Stay within your estimated calorie requirements each day (see page 36).*

3. **Nutrient Density**—*Choose food that contains plenty of nutrients, such as vitamins and minerals.*

4. **Moderation**—*Try not to consume too much of any one food.*

5. **Variety**—*Eat a wide selection of healthy foods from the major food groups.*

Practice

Before you go to bed each night, think about what you will eat the next day. Set your alarm clock 15 minutes early so that you will have time to start your day with breakfast and still have time to pack a nutritious lunch and mid-afternoon snack.

Nutritional Health

*R*esearch has revealed that you consistently lose more weight and make healthier food choices when you write down what you eat and the amount you eat each day.

Practice

Keep a food journal. Buy a calorie counting book and a small notebook. Keep a record of the food you eat. Use it to discover areas that need improvement, as well as healthy habits to continue. Don't forget to write down the calories you consume in the beverages you drink. The extra calories you consume in beverages do little to satisfy hunger, but add to your caloric intake just the same.

*C*ertian foods have been linked to reducing
the risks of developing particular diseases.

Practice

Make an effort to consume at least five
foods from this list each day. Be
mindful of the recommended portion
and serving sizes of each.

- **Blueberries**—contain an antioxidant,
  which helps reduce the risk of cancer
- **Tomatoes**—contain lycopene, which
  also helps to reduce the risk of developing prostate cancer
- **Fish**—contains omega-3 fatty acids,
  which lowers risk of atherosclerosis
  and decreases the risk of heart disease
- **Spinach**—contains lutein, an antioxidant, and also an excellent source
  of calcium and folate, which are
  especially important in a woman's diet
- **Oatmeal**—helps to reduce cholesterol
  levels and decreases the risk of cardiovascular disease

(continued on next page)

(continued from previous page)

- **Nuts**—high in vitamin E, which reduces the risk of cardiovascular disease and helps protect red blood cells

- **Garlic**—contains allyl sulfides, which facilitate a process that excretes carcinogens, or cancer-causing agents

- **Green tea**—helps to maintain blood sugar to moderate levels and reduces the risk of cardiovascular disease

- **Olive oil**—a source of monounsaturated fat, which helps to improve the HDL levels, or "good" cholesterol in your blood

- **Red wine, red grapes or grape juice**—contains flavonoids, which decrease the risk of heart disease

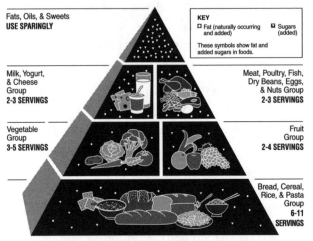

Food Guide Pyramid
A Guide to Daily Food Choices

Fats, Oils, & Sweets
USE SPARINGLY

KEY
□ Fat (naturally occurring and added)   ◪ Sugars (added)
These symbols show fat and added sugars in foods.

Milk, Yogurt, & Cheese Group
2-3 SERVINGS

Meat, Poultry, Fish, Dry Beans, Eggs, & Nuts Group
2-3 SERVINGS

Vegetable Group
3-5 SERVINGS

Fruit Group
2-4 SERVINGS

Bread, Cereal, Rice, & Pasta Group
6-11 SERVINGS

Source: U.S. Department of Agriculture / U.S. Department of Health and Human Services. Note: Periodic revisions can be expected in the Food Guide Pyramid as the USDA evaluates ongoing research in the area of nutrition.

Practice

Use this as a general guide for making healthy food choices. The number of servings that is right for you will depend on the number of calories you need. Try to consume at least the lowest recommended number of servings for each category to ensure your body is getting all the nutrients it needs.

*M*ajor Nutrients:

- **Carbohydrates** are the body's primary source of fuel. The brain relies entirely on carbohydrates for energy.

- **Proteins** serve the body by providing energy, supporting growth and repairing body structures such as the skin, muscles, tendons, bones and organs.

- **Fat** is necessary in transporting other nutrients in the body. It also plays a vital role in the growth and development of the body.

Practice

Avoid a diet that completely eliminates any one of these categories.

Nutritional Health

he ever increasing portion sizes available when eating out can skew our idea of what actual recommended portions sizes really look like. The major reason individuals gain weight is simply that they eat too much in comparison to their activity level.

Practice

Learn to monitor and control food serving sizes. Measure and weigh the food you eat for a few days so that you will learn what a correct portion size looks like. Soon you will be able to control your portions by simply looking at the amount of food on your plate.

Examples of recommended serving sizes:

Breads, Cereals, Rice, and Pasta
- 1 slice of bread
- $1/2$ cup cooked cereal, rice or pasta
- $1/2$ bun
- bagel
- English muffin

(continued on next page)

(continued from previous page)

Fruit
- 1 medium piece of fruit
- $1/2$ cup chopped, cooked or canned fruit
- $1/2$ cup of juice

Vegetables
- 1 cup raw leafy vegetables
- $1/2$ cup all other vegetables (cooked or chopped raw)

Milk, Yogurt, and Cheese
- 1 cup milk or yogurt
- $1^1/2$ ounces natural cheese
- 2 ounces processed cheese
- $1/2$ cup ice cream or frozen yogurt

Meat, Poultry, Fish, Dry Beans, Eggs, and Nuts
- 2 to 3 ounces lean cooked meat, poultry or fish
- $1/2$ cup cooked beans
- 1 egg or 2 egg whites
- $1/4$ cup tofu
- 2 tablespoons of seeds, nuts, or peanut butter as 1 ounce of meat

Fats, Oils, and Sweets—Eat sparingly!

If you eat right and exercise, you will reap the rewards of a healthier and more attractive body.

Practice

Focus on the health benefits of a balanced diet, rather than the aesthetic benefits. Adapt a life-long eating plan, rather than a diet for weight loss.

No food should be labeled as "bad." All foods can fit into a balanced diet as long as moderation and portion sizes are considered.

Practice

Don't deny yourself! Allow yourself to indulge in your favorite craving—within reason. By allowing yourself a small piece of chocolate each day, or dessert on the weekends, you will decrease the risk of binge eating. Because you are not fixated on the foods you can't eat, you will be more satisfied with healthy choices throughout the day.

*M*aking *healthy food choices is among the most effective actions you can take to be productive and feel your best.*

Practice

Become familiar with the various sections of a food label so that you will understand the nutritional value of the food you eat. Do not be misguided by inaccurate information. When in doubt, check with your doctor, a registered dietitian, the County Cooperative Extension Service, the nutrition department at a university or community college, or professional health organizations. Be cautious of claims that promise quick fixes or miraculous cures or results.

(continued on next page)

(continued from previous page)

$\mathcal{R}$eading food labels

Serving size:
Represents the amount people actually eat. If you double the serving listed, be sure to double the amount of nutrients and calories consumed.

Calories:
Look here to see how a serving of this food adds to your daily total of calories needed.

List of nutrients:
This section covers the most important nutrients by listing how many grams of each are in one serving.

Vitamins and minerals:
Your goal is to reach 100% of each for the day. You will need a combination of foods in order to acheive this.

Nutrition Facts

Serving Size ½ cup (114g)
Servings Per Container 4

Amount Per Serving

Calories 90   Calories from Fat 30

	% Daily Value*
Total Fat 3g	**5%**
Saturated Fat 0g	**0%**
Cholesterol 0mg	**0%**
Sodium 300mg	**13%**
Total Carbohydrate 13g	**4%**
Dietary Fiber 3g	**12%**
Sugars 3g	
Protein 3g	

Vitamin A 80%	•	Vitamin C 60%
Calcium 4%	•	Iron 4%

*Percent Daily Values are based on a 2,000 calorie diet. Your daily values may be higher or lower depending on your calorie needs:

	Calories:	2,000	2,500
Total Fat	Less than	65g	80g
Sat Fat	Less than	20g	25g
Cholesterol	Less than	300mg	300mg
Sodium	Less than	2,400mg	2,400mg
Total Carbohydrate		300g	375g
Dietary Fiber		25g	30g

Calories per gram:
Fat 9 • Carbohydrate 4 • Protein 4

Calories from fat:
Try to limit the number of calories from fat. Choose foods that get no more than 30% of their calories from fat.

% Daily values:
Percentages represent how this food fits into the overall daily intake of calories. Use this section to determine if it contributes a little or a lot of a certain nutrient.

Daily values:
These are listed for people who consume 2,000 or 2,500 calories each day. If your caloric intake is higher, your % daily values will be also. If your caloric intake is lower, your % daily values will be also.

*U*nderstanding *popular food claims and descriptions is essential to eating right.*

Practice

In order to reduce the amount of fat, sugar, and/or calories in your diet, look for foods that carry the appropriate claims.

Fat-free: Less than 0.5 grams of fat per serving

Low fat: 3 grams or less of fat per serving

Less, Fewer, or Reduced: 25% less of a given nutrient or calories than the comparison food

Low calorie: 40 calories or less per serving

Light (fat): 50% or less fat than the comparison food

Light (calories): $1/3$ fewer calories than the comparison food

Not eating enough can trick your body into thinking it is starving. Then your metabolism drops and your body begins to conserve energy (as stored fat).

Practice

Start each day with breakfast and eat at regular intervals throughout the day. Never allow yourself to get too hungry.

Nutritional Health

Snacks are a great way to decrease hunger and re-energize you until your next meal.

Practice

Choose snacks that combine carbo-hydrates for energy, and protein and fiber to help you feel full longer. Try a cup of vegetable soup, cereal with skim milk and fruit, or sliced apples or celery dipped in peanut butter.

Your weight in pounds divided by two equals the number of ounces of water you need to consume in order to supply your body with the proper amount of hydration.

Example: 150 pounds ÷ 2 = 75 ounces
Note: 8 ounces = one cup

Practice

Keep a water bottle with you to sip from throughout the day. Try to substitute water for just one sugary soda a day, and you will save enough calories to lose one pound of fat per month.

W̶ater benefits the body by:
- *Metabolizing stored fat*
- *Carrying nutrients to the cells*
- *Providing the basic foundation of all body fluids*
- *Removing waste*
- *Suppressing appetite*
- *Decreasing fluid retention*
- *Lubricating and cushioning joints*

Practice

Drink up! The easiest way to tell if you are adequately hydrated is to check the color and quantity of your urine. If it is clear or light colored, your body is getting the water it needs. If it is dark, you need to drink more fluids (see page 53 for guidelines).

Simple Fitness
For Your Mind

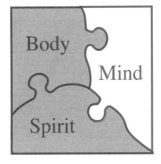

Intellectual Health

Just like the muscles in your body, the brain thrives on the motto of "Use it, or lose it."

Practice

Stimulate your brain by making it work beyond its normal routine. Try brushing your hair with the opposite hand. Take an alternate route home from work. Work a crossword puzzle. Don't let your thought processes get stuck in a rut!

*R*eading, learning new vocabulary words, and solving problems exercise the brain. These exercises help to create more neurotransmitters in the brain and stronger dendrites, which allow thought patterns to connect more efficiently.

Practice

Work those brain cells. Stimulate brain activity. Read an entry from a dictionary or go to www.dictionary.com and learn a new word daily. Obtain a book list from a public library or retail book store and set a goal to read a certain number of books a year. Learn new vocabulary words each month from *Reader's Digest* "It Pays to Enrich Your Word Power."

*W*hat you did is not important. What you learned from it is.

Practice

Do not be afraid to try new things. Use every experience as a learning opportunity. Embrace a life of questions. Seek answers. Research facts. Draw conclusions.

"First say to yourself what you would be, then do what you have to do."

—Epicetus

Practice

First, plan your goal. Next, plan your strategy. Consider dividing the goal into mini-goals and plan dates for attainment. Research every aspect of your goal. No goal is ever too lofty. Let your goal be a vision or dream that becomes reality.

Intellectual Health

*R*esearch has demonstrated the many health benefits of listening to music including improved memory, logic, creativity, and standardized test scores, as well as less stress, anxiety, and depression.

Practice

Listen to music, relax and de-stress. Find comfort in soft piano music or your favorite compact disk. Music suggestion: Louis Armstrong's "It's a Wonderful World."

*P*erspective is based on one's experiences. Broaden your perspective by seeking to gain knowledge or experience in a subject you know nothing about.

Practice

Choose a subject in which you would like to be more knowledgeable. This subject could range from car mechanics to a foreign language to current events. Pursue the facts through the Internet, a bookstore, or your local library. You can become the specialist about subjects that interest you. Feed on information.

Memorization helps stimulate the mind and comes in handy for references in conversation.

Practice

Memorize your favorite poems, Bible verses, or quotes. Go over the words numerous times until they are familiar and easy to recite. Practice memorizing phone numbers. Always associate people's names with descriptive objects. This will help you remember names more readily.

"*Life is a series of experiences, each one of which makes us bigger, even though sometimes it is hard to realize this. For the world was built to develop character, and we must learn that the setbacks and grief which we endure help us in our marching onward.*"

—Henry Ford

Practice

Realize that setbacks are growing experiences that allow you to reflect on what has happened and seek an alternative plan. Never compromise your values in this endeavor.

Intellectual Health

*R*esearch *has revealed chewing gum stimulates brain activity by producing a calming effect.*

Practice

Chew gum when you take a test or need to concentrate for a long period of time.

Intellectual Health

Wellness is a conscious effort to make positive decisions about life. It is choosing to be healthy and performing tasks that enhance your quality of life.

Practice

Change the things you can, accept the things you cannot. Live for the present and future, learn from your past. Choose to be lighter about life, go with the flow and be thankful for at least five things each morning. Don't be satisfied to feel OK. Choose to be happy, vibrant and in control. Remember you have choices, make wise ones. When making decisions, read all the information you can about the subject you are deciding upon.

Social Health

*S*tudies show that the more socially active a person is, the better their memory.

Practice

Be socially active. Call your family. Email old friends. Remember and acknowledge birthdays and special dates of friends and family. Develop new friendships. Be positive and keep a smile on your face. The best way to enter a room of people is to enter with a smile. Then everyone wants to get to know you.

Social Health

*S*ocial situations can have a positive influence on your personal health choices.

Practice

Start a supper club that focuses on health. Get together with three or four other couples and share a healthy meal. Let each person be in charge of a different course that is easy and healthy. Share the recipes and start a file. Enjoy the conversation. Finish off the evening with a relaxing walk. If you have children, teach them healthy practices by including them in the event.

"*H*appiness is not a destination. It is a method of life."

—Burton Hills

Practice

Smile at five or more people daily. Choose to be happy—work at it. Think good thoughts. Do good things. Look for the positive. Appreciate the good in people. Do not ignore the people around you as you strive toward your dreams. Enjoy and appreciate those who are the landmarks along your journey. Make a list of your blessings. Reflect daily on them. Concentrate on the positive aspects of life.

Establishing a sense of community increases your health and happiness. The encouragement of friends who have similar interests supports and strengthens your health goals and helps you to develop and attain positive health actions.

Practice

If your social circle is small and time limits your ability to get involved in local or church events, try the Internet. Many websites sponsor chats and forums related to special interests. Develop a sense of community by chatting with others who have similar interests as you. Many wellness sites have chat rooms. Be selective about the sites you explore.

*T*he earth provides us with so many wonderful resources—don't take her for granted.

Practice

Help out your environment. Join a volunteer organization or organize your own group that will strive to clean up a local stream or park. Not only will you provide a service to your community's environment, you will be filled with pride and a sense of accomplishment by making a difference. Don't forget to recycle. Help keep our resources to their maximum benefit for society.

Social Health

Social interaction does not necessarily involve other humans. Having a pet has been shown to:

- *Lower blood pressure*
- *Aid in stress management*
- *Lower incidence of minor health problems*
- *Improve psychological well-being*
- *Reduce loneliness and isolation*
- *Reduce heart attack death*

Practice

Consider adopting a pet. If you already have a pet, take advantage of the potential health benefits and spend time walking, petting, or playing with your pet. It's good for you!

*P*eople *who workout together and share the same fitness goals are more likely to be successful.*

Practice

Join an exercise group. Try an exercise class at a local gym. Join a walking/jogging club. If there are no clubs of this sort in your area, or you would rather be surrounded with people you already know, head up your own group. Recruit friends, co-workers, or fellow church members. Meet three times a week for an evening walk, train for a 5K race together, or workout to an exercise video at someone's house. Encourage and motivate each other. Celebrate achievements. Be accountable to a minimum of two people for your daily workouts. Social support systems of family and/or friends help you to achieve health goals you could not reach alone. Set a convenient time for your daily workouts that enables you to visit with a friend also.

*T*he well-being of the mind and body are intimately intertwined with each other. What happens in the kidneys, pancreas, or liver can affect the brain's activity. Consequently, disorders of the mind can signal biochemical disturbances that interrupt normal functions throughout the entire body.

Practice

Remember, the mind and body are not separate. Don't "stress out" over small incidences. This can put your body in turmoil. Take deep breaths, relax, and think of constructive ways to deal with problems.

"Believe in yourself! Have faith in your abilities! Without a humble but reasonable confidence in your own powers you cannot be successful or happy."
—Norman Vincent Peale

Practice

Do not start a project that you don't believe in. Gain respect from your peers through your confidence in what is right. The first step in confidence is being well prepared. You will make mistakes on your way to success; look at these as teaching tools. Know your limitations but focus on your strengths and assets.

*S*etting goals increases the likelihood of accomplishment. The goals we set—and the motivating beliefs about these goals—direct our lives and give it purpose. Keep your goals attainable but also worthy of your time and efforts.

Practice

Set goals. Get rid of "hang-ups" that tend to bombard you with worry. Think through these strategies for possible change. Think about what is really important to you and make a list. Next, write down specific goals and mini goals that pertain to these interests. Allow ample time to develop goals in these specific areas. Be flexible and regroup if goals change as your priorities change.

*R*esearch shows that people with positive personalities meet goals more readily and realize their hopes and dreams more often.

Practice

Think optimistically; always hope and dream. Be prepared to meet your life's dream every day, any time. Be confident and poised, always presenting your best self. Focus on the positive in every situation. Do not allow yourself to get caught up in the negatives, which will only steal your joy.

Cortisol, a hormone released in the brain when you are stressed, destroys brain cells and may form plaque within the blood vessels which may cause heart disease and strokes.

Practice

Practice relaxation techniques to reduce stress. Simply tense and relax specific muscle groups, moving from your head all the way down to your toes. Visualize your favorite relaxing setting. Take a minimum of three 10-minute time-outs a day in which you clear your mind and seek to relax your body. This exercise may save your life.

Pamper yourself. Everyone deserves a day off. Prioritize your weekly schedule allowing time for you. Studies show people are more productive if they have a "reward" or a goal to look forward to. A morning, an afternoon, an hour or a day just for you—what a prize!

Practice

What do you really enjoy doing that you feel you never have time to do? Do your favorite things—eat chocolate, read a great book, give yourself a manicure, lie on the couch and watch old movies, take a hike down your favorite trail, take a long, hot, soothing bath. Take the time and enjoy.

*Selfishness turns life into a burden.
Unselfishness turns burdens into life!*

Practice

Embrace a life of service to others.
Perform unselfish acts of love in every
situation. Volunteer work provides
wonderful help for society and gives
you a sense of peace and fulfillment.
Volunteer at a local library to help
adults learn to read. Volunteer for a
service agency such as the American
Heart Association, American Cancer
Society, American Red Cross, or one of
the many others.

Emotional Health

The ability to experience and express a wide range of human emotions and to steer those emotions in a positive direction is an asset.

Practice

Recognize your feelings and emotions.
Express them in a positive manner.
Do not allow unhealthy thoughts such
as prolonged grief or guilt to make you
habitually sad or bitter. Choose to be
happy. It is your decision.

*E*motional intelligence is the capacity for recognizing our own feelings and those of others, for motivating ourselves, and for managing emotions in ourselves and our relationships.

Practice

Think before you act. Recognize other people's feelings. Try to understand why someone is saying or doing a particular thing. Look at each situation from someone else's point of view. Never judge another.

*L*ife *is too short not to embrace special occasions. Be creative and initiate "moments to remember."*

Practice

Celebrate everything! Birthdays, report card days, raises, anniversaries . . . there are many days that can be celebrated. Plan something wonderful to help celebrate all great days. Hang balloons, enjoy a special meal, use an "it's your special day plate," go on a picnic. Everyone likes to feel special. Don't let life go by without complimenting someone by planning a special celebration in their honor. You will be making memories.

Never look at what you have lost. Look at what you have left.

Practice

Concentrate on everything that is good
and enjoyable. Accept the things
you cannot change and dwell on the
pleasurable things in your life.

*L*aughter relaxes the entire body and burns 78 times as many calories as when you are sitting or lying still. *Laughter also produces more T-cells, an important component of a healthy immune system.*

Practice

Lighten up. Laugh frequently and vigorously!

Recalling positive scenes and situations when facing stressful times or moments of depression can have a calming effect.

Practice

Imprint in your mind the images and sounds from scenes that give you a euphoric feeling. Watch a sunset from a seashore, gaze at bright city lights from a high mountain peak, step into new snow on a crisp, glittery winter morning, hold a new born baby, peer at the stars in the black sky on a clear night, sit in the white sand on a beach while listening to the roar of the waves. Proclamations of this wonderful world are everywhere. Look for them. Remember them. When facing stressful times, visualize these moments of wonder.

Simple Fitness
For Your Spirit

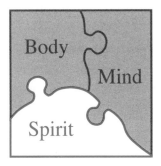

"Prayer is a powerful and effectual worry-remover. Men and women who have learned to pray with childlike sincerity, literally talking to, and communing with the Heavenly Father, are in possession of the great secret, whereby they can cast their care upon God, knowing that He careth for us. A clear conscious is a great step toward barricading the mind against neuroticism."

> —Dr. William Sadler's advice to physicians on how to pinpoint the cause of people's trouble, from the book *None of These Diseases.*

Practice

Always be aware of these words:

Peace I leave with you, my peace I give unto you: not as the world giveth, give I unto you. Let not your heart be troubled, neither let it be afraid.

John 14:27 (KJV)

*D*o not be anxious about anything, but in
everything, by prayer and petition, with
thanksgiving, present your request to God.

Phillipians 4:6 (NIV)

Practice

If you are burdened with worry and
stress, ask God to guide you down the
path that is best, so that His will is
done. The act of worrying takes time
and energy—time and energy that could
be better spent in prayer, followed by
patience or action prompted by God.

Consider how the lilies grow. They do not labor or spin. Yet I tell you, not even Solomon in all his splendor was dressed as one of these.

Luke 12:27 (NIV)

Practice

Let nature be a part of your meditation practice. Focus on nature as a way to rid your body of stress. Consider how the simplicity and peacefulness of the lilies surpassed the praise of worldly things.

*T*ake *my yoke upon you, and learn of me;
for I am meek and lowly in heart: and ye shall
find rest unto your souls.*

Matthew 11:29 (KJV)

Practice

As you overcome obstacles while you press toward your goals, remember to stay humble. For it is with God's help that you are able to progress. Do not allow your triumphs to intimidate others, but use these triumphs as examples to help others learn of the strength they too possess.

"It's not the load that breaks you down, it's the way you carry it."

—Anonymous

Even youths grow tired and weary, and young men stumble and fall; but those who hope in the Lord will renew their strength. They will soar on wings like eagles; they will run and not grow weary, they will walk and not be faint.

Isaiah 40:30-31 (NIV)

Practice

Don't grow weak in waiting for the Lord. He will give you strength to withstand your trials and promises the faithful rewards in spiritual prosperity.

The wicked flee when no one is pursuing, but the righteous are bold as a lion.

Proverbs 28:1 (NAS)

Practice

Be courageous in times of trial. Your righteous living in the Lord will go before you, beside you, and behind you. He will enable you to be strong and bold to glorify Him.

*H*e that hath no rule over his own spirit is
*like a city that is broken down, and without
walls.*

Proverbs 25:28 (KJV)

Practice

You and God are the only ones who
have control over your spirit. Know
that God loves you and always wants
what is best for you. Do not let others
bring you down. Other people do not
have the power to upset you, anger you,
or discourage you—only you can allow
that to happen. Stay in control with
God's Guidance.

"Be faithful in the little things, for in them our strength lies."

—Mother Teresa

Practice

View each accomplishment, whether it be big or small, as a great achievement. Have faith in yourself and in your abilities. Begin making a list of your accomplishments and let your confidence build as your list grows.

A good name is better than precious ointment. . .

Ecclesiastes 7:1 (KJV)

Practice

Your name is what you make of it.
Write down the things you would like
for people to think about when they
hear your name. Do you live up to your
list? Strive to be the person that you
want associated with your name.

*N*ow faith is the substance of things hoped
for, the evidence of things not seen.

Hebrews 11:1 (KJV)

Practice

Through God, all things are possible.
Have faith in God, and you can have
faith in all things. Think of your goals,
the things you hope to accomplish,
and through faith know that they are
possible.

*A*re you imprisoned by the desire of want?
*(Just one more thing, one more car, one more
television, a larger house, etc.)*

Practice

The psalmist David relays to us the
secret of satisfaction:

*The Lord is my Shepherd; I shall
not want.*

Psalms 23:1 (KJV)

Be joyful always . . . give thanks in all circumstances . . .

1 Thessalonians 5:16, 18 (NIV)

Practice

When the day gets long or times get tough, take a moment and write down at least ten things you can be thankful for. Include any blessing you wish; no blessing is too small. You will then realize how blessed you really are.

... *Let us lay aside every weight ... let us run with patience the race that is set before us.*

Hebrews 12:1 (KJV)

Practice

Setbacks will happen, accept it and move on. Do not let setbacks in life hinder your happiness and lead you off course. Give your cares over to the Lord.

"Yesterday is gone.
Tomorrow has not yet come.
We have only today. Let us begin."

—Mother Teresa

Practice

Believe in today. Don't wait until tomorrow—or the first of next week, month, or year—to start striving toward your goals. Don't focus your thoughts on failures in the past. Set your sights on dreams and know that you are not alone. Ask God to lead you day by day on the journey to accomplishments. Write down the step you need to accomplish today in order to make your dreams come true. A small step each day will put you closer and closer to your goal.

*C*ast all your anxiety on Him because he cares for you.

1 Peter 5:7 (NIV)

Practice

Don't be fretful. God knows your every thought and need. He will comfort you and strengthen you in times of trouble. Give your worries to God in prayer.

Cease striving and know that I am God . . .

Psalm 46:10 (NAS)

Practice

The Lord is our refuge. He is our help
in time of trouble. When the Lord Jesus
is our strength, we will not fear nor be
anxious. Claim it!

I will put my trust in Him . . .

Hebrews 2:13 (NIV)

Practice

Trust in the Lord. He is working for your good. Patiently wait for His power and might.

"No peace lies in the future which is not hidden in this present instant. Take peace."

—Fra Giovanni Giocondo, 1513

Practice

While working toward achieving your goals, be happy with who you are along the way. When you doubt yourself, think of just one positive attribute and act upon it. If that positive attribute is being a friendly person, then make an effort to smile at each person you meet. Always find peace in the positive.

You alone are the Lord. You made the heavens, even the highest heavens, and all their starry host, the earth and all that is on it, the seas and all that is in them. You give life to everything, and the multitudes of heaven worship you.

Nehemiah 9:6 (NIV)

Practice

Allow yourself frequent opportunities to appreciate the beauty of God's creation. Take a nature walk, or stop and marvel at the beauty of the flowers and trees you pass by regularly.

*F*or since the creation of the world, God's invisible qualities, his eternal power and divine nature, have been clearly seen being understood from what has been made, so that men were without excuse.

Romans 1:20 (NIV)

Practice

Focus on the greatness of God's abilities by observing nature. Notice that every natural process has a purpose and, in turn, affects its surroundings. You, too, are evidence of God's greatness. As part of His creation, you have a purpose that will impact all that surrounds you.

*For I know the plans I have for you . . .
plans to prosper you and not harm you,
plans to give you hope and a future.*

Jeremiah 29:11 (NIV)

Practice

Trust in the Lord, that He is working in
your life for good. Though circumstances
may seem tough sometimes, the Lord
will see you through and give you a
bright future. Believe.

*D*o It Anyway

People are often unreasonable,
illogical and self-centered;
Forgive them anyway.

If you are kind, people may accuse you
of selfish, ulterior motives;
Be kind anyway.

If you are successful, you will win some
false friends, and some true enemies;
Succeed anyway.

If you are honest and frank,
people may cheat you;
Be honest and frank anyway.

What you spend years building,
someone could destroy overnight;
Build anyway.

If you find serenity and happiness,
they will be jealous;
Be happy anyway.

The good you do today,
people will often forget tomorrow;
Do good anyway.

Give the world the best you have,
and it may not be enough;
Give the world the best you've got anyway.

You see, in the final analysis,
it is between you and God;
It is never between you and them anyway.

—Anonymous

Bibliography

Delta Society. (n.d.). *Healthy reasons to have a pet.* Retrieved December 19, 2003, from http://www.deltasociety.org/ dsc020.htm

Escott-Stump, S., Mahan, L.K. (2000). *Krause's Food Nutrition, and Diet Therapy* (10th ed.). Philadelphia, PA: W.B.Saunders.

Goleman, D. (1998). *Working with Emotional Intelligence.* New York: Bantam Books.

Holy Bible. (1984). *The New Scofield Study Bible,* New International Version. New York: Oxford University.

Holy Bible. (1972). *Old and New Testaments in the King James Version.* Nashville: Thomas Nelson.

Holy Bible. (1977). *The Starter Study Bible,* New American Standard Version. Iowa Falls, IA: World Bible.

Insel, P., Roth, W. (1996). *Core Concepts in Health.* Boston: McGraw-Hill.

Keen, C.L., Steinberg, F.M. (2003). *Cocoa and Chocolate Flavonoids: Implications for Cardiovascular Health.* Journal of the American Dietetic Association, 103(2), 215-223.

Khalsa, D.S. (1999). *Brain Longevity.* New York: Warner Books.

Lemonick, M.D. (2003, Jan. 20). "Your Mind, Your Body." *Time* Special Issue, 161(3), pg. 63 Bearden, M.M.

Lucado, M. (2001). *Traveling Light.* Dallas, TX: Word Publishing.

McMillen, S.I. (1963). *None of these Diseases.* New Jersey: Fleming H. Revel.

Rolfes, S.R. (1996). *Understanding Nutrition.* St. Paul, MN: West.

Schuler, R. (1996). *The Be Happy Attitudes.* Nashville, TN: W Publishing Group.

Seaward, B.L. (2001). *Health of the Human Spirit.* Boston: Allyn and Bacon.

Smith, H.W. (1998). *The Christian's Secret of a Happy Life.* Uhrichsville, OH: Barbour.

Surgeon General's Office. (1996). "A Report of the Surgeon General: Physical Activity and Health." U.S. Department of Health and Human Services.

Swindoll, C.R. (1990). *Stress Fractures.* Portland, OR: Multnomah Press.

University of California, Berkley. (2003, Jan.). *Wellness Made Easy.* The Newsletter of Nutrition, Fitness, and Self-Care, 19(4).

Vass. S. (1989). *Laugh Your Way to Good Health!* Atlanta: HMR Publication Group.

About the Authors

Amanda Conrad holds a Bachelor of Science degree in Physical Education, with a concentration in Fitness Management, and a second degree in Human Sciences, with a concentration in Food and Nutrition, both from Mississippi State University. She is currently completing a dietetic internship through the University of Delaware.

Conrad is a practicing National Strength and Conditioning Association (NSCA) certified personal trainer and Aerobic and Fitness Association of America (AFAA) certified fitness instructor. She firmly believes that those who desire physical fitness and improved health respond better to a simple approach.

She and her husband, Mann, reside in Starkville, Mississippi.

Dr. Joyce Yates is Associate Professor, Emma Ody Pohl Endowed Chair and coordinator of the graduate program in health education in the Division of Health and Kinesiology at Mississippi University for Women. She has taught health and physical education in higher education for over 20 years. Dr. Yates, along with MUW graduate students, has enjoyed putting time and effort into the health education program "Commit To Be Fit" for the MUW campus and Columbus community.

Dr. Yates received a Bachelor of Science degree from the University of Mississippi, and a Master of Science degree and a Doctor of Education degree from Mississippi State University. During her undergraduate education at the University of Mississippi, she was a member of the first Ole Miss women's intercollegiate basketball and tennis teams. Dr. Yates lives in Eupora, Mississippi, with her husband, Bill. They have three children, Claire of Nashville, Tennessee, and Tripp and Trent of Eupora.